DEFEATING STOMACH ULCER WITH EXPERT GUIDANCE

Ultimate Solution Handbook For Patients, Guardians Or Family To Understand, Manage, Treat, Prevent, Reverse Symptoms And Live Well

DR. POTTER WHITLEY

Copyright © 2023 by Dr. Potter Whitley

DISCLAIMER:

This book's contents are meant to be used solely for informative purposes. The information should not be used as a replacement for expert medical advice, diagnosis, or care.

The information contained in this book is accurate and reliable, having been verified by the author to the best of his ability. Nevertheless, the author disclaims all express and implied representations and warranties regarding the availability, correctness, appropriateness, completeness, and reliability of the material provided here. You bear full responsibility for any reliance you may have on such material.

For informational purposes, this book may make reference to or mention of certain people, things, websites, organizations, or other names. The author has no connection to, endorsement from, or recommendation for these organizations. The author's approval or validation is not implied by the inclusion of these references.

Any direct, indirect, incidental, special, or consequential damages resulting from using or not being able to use the material in this book are not covered by the author's liability policy. For medical advice and counsel particular to their circumstances, readers are advised to check with experienced healthcare specialists.

The content, materials, and information in this book are subject to change at any time without prior notice, at the author's discretion. The text may contain errors or omissions for which the author is not responsible.

By reading this book, you understand and accept the conditions of this disclaimer.

THE REASON BEHIND THIS BOOK

In the field of digestive health, "Defeating STOMACH ULCER With Expert Guidance" is a shining light of empowerment and knowledge. This in-depth manual explores the complex terrain of stomach ulcers and provides a complete method that enables people to take control of their health. Readers have a thorough grasp of stomach ulcers through a thorough investigation of causes, symptoms, and diagnosis, providing the groundwork for making well-informed decisions.

The strength of this work comes from its dedication to elucidating the scientific aspects of stomach ulcers, including the roles played by stress, genetics, gastric acid, and Helicobacter pylori infection. These sections provide vital insights and expert counsel, building upon this scientific foundation. To receive an accurate diagnosis and individualized treatment regimens, readers are encouraged to interact with healthcare specialists, underscoring the significance of seeking professional assistance.

This handbook offers a wide range of treatment alternatives, from traditional prescription drugs to surgical procedures and complementary therapies. One really good section is on nutrition and diet, with helpful advice on how to prevent stomach ulcers by eating sensibly and staying hydrated.

This book goes beyond simple medical recommendations to address stress management, acknowledging the significant influence of stress on stomach ulcers. The story skillfully incorporates practical methods, mind-body exercises, and resilient lifestyle strategies to provide readers with a comprehensive arsenal for healing.

This book stands out for its commitment to preventative measures and comprehensive methods. To promote gut health, readers are taken through the integration of mind, body, and spirit while learning about herbal medicines, yoga, and meditation. The path to preventing recurrence is meticulously mapped out, emphasizing follow-up care, long-term maintenance, and the development of individualized preventive programs.

One of the main themes is navigating the difficulties associated with managing stomach ulcers, including emotional elements, side effects of treatment, and the critical function of support networks. The plot is inspired by real-life success stories and testimonies, which turns this book into a motivating and uplifting read.

"Defeating STOMACH ULCER With Expert Guidance" ultimately goes beyond the confines of a standard health book. It serves as a road map for empowerment, encouraging readers to take responsibility for their health, develop all-encompassing well-being plans, and work toward raising awareness. For individuals with stomach ulcers, this book offers a ray of hope and wisdom because of its upbeat tone and insightful material.

TABLE OF CONTENT

CHAPTER ONE

UNDERSTANDING STOMACH ULCERS
How Do Stomach Ulcers Occur?

Peptic ulcers, another name for stomach ulcers, are open sores that appear on the inside of the small intestine or the lining of the stomach. The lining that protects the stomach and intestines from the corrosive effects of stomach acids is eroding, which causes these ulcers. The bacterium Helicobacter pylori (H. pylori) or long-term use of nonsteroidal anti-inflammatory medicines (NSAIDs) are frequently cited as the main causes of stomach ulcers. Acidic digestive juices can pierce the delicate lining when the protective mucous layer is breached, resulting in the formation of ulcers.

The size and severity of stomach ulcers can vary, from tiny, superficial sores to larger, deeper lesions that, if left untreated, could result in serious consequences.

There is a wide range of symptoms that can be connected to stomach ulcers, and people may feel different amounts of pain or discomfort. Comprehending the fundamental reasons and contributing elements is essential for efficient mitigation and handling.

Reasons and Danger Elements

The bacterium H is the main culprit behind stomach ulcers. pylori. This bacterium makes the stomach more vulnerable to acid injury by degrading the mucous membrane that coats the stomach. Additionally, by preventing the synthesis of chemicals that shield the stomach lining, long-term use of NSAIDs like aspirin and ibuprofen might hasten the formation of ulcers.

Additional risk factors encompass smoking, binge drinking enormous amounts of alcohol, and specific medical diseases including Zollinger-Ellison syndrome. While stress and spicy foods were formerly thought to be important contributors, new medical research indicates that they may not be the direct causes, even though they may exacerbate symptoms.

Effective treatment for stomach ulcers requires early detection. Tests to identify H may be used as diagnostic techniques, as well as endoscopy, which involves inserting a flexible tube equipped with a camera into the digestive tract to view ulcers. pylori infection.

Signs and Prognosis

The symptoms of stomach ulcers can range widely, from minor discomfort to excruciating pain. Symptoms such as nausea, bloating, burning in the stomach, and fullness are common. In more serious situations, people may throw up, lose weight without knowing why, or have dark, tarry stools, which are signs of bleeding ulcers.

A complete medical history review, a physical examination, and several diagnostic procedures are all necessary for making a diagnosis. Tests for H can be performed on the blood, stool, and breath. pylori infection, although imaging tests such as CT or X-rays can show the presence and severity of ulcers. For precise diagnosis, endoscopy is still an essential tool for direct imaging and biopsy of ulcerated regions.

Various Kinds Of Stomach Ulcers

Based on their site and underlying causes, stomach ulcers can be divided into different categories. Duodenal ulcers form in the top portion of the small intestine, whereas gastric ulcers originate in the lining of the stomach. Comprehending these differences is essential to customizing treatment strategies.

Additionally, there are two types of stomach ulcers: acute and chronic. Generally superficial, acute ulcers can heal on their own with the right medicine and lifestyle modifications. On the other hand, chronic ulcers are deeper and can need longer, more thorough treatments.

In summary, knowing the nature, causes, symptoms, and types of stomach ulcers is essential to have a thorough grasp of them. Promoting overall digestive health and well-being, and controlling and preventing complications related to stomach ulcers requires early detection and proper medical action.

CHAPTER TWO

THE SCIENCE OF ULCERS IN THE STOMACH
Gastric Acid: Its Function

Gastric acid is an essential part of digestion, which is facilitated by the intricate function of the stomach. The gastric glands in the lining of the stomach secrete gastric acid, which is mainly hydrochloric acid. Its primary job is to disintegrate food particles into smaller, easier-to-digest parts. Although stomach acid is necessary for digestion, an imbalance in its production or management can result in several gastrointestinal problems, such as ulcers in the stomach.

Peptic ulcers, another name for stomach ulcers, are caused by erosion of the stomach's protective lining, which exposes the underlying tissues to the damaging effects of gastric acid. Ulcers may arise as a result of a compromised mucosal barrier or excessive stomach acid production. Developing successful management and prevention measures for stomach ulcers requires a thorough understanding of the delicate balance of gastric acid production and its effects on the stomach lining.

To lessen acidity and encourage the healing of tissues that have been ulcerated, researchers have looked at the use of drugs to control stomach acid levels. To regulate acid secretion, proton pump inhibitors (PPIs) and histamine receptor blockers are frequently administered. Achieving a balance is crucial, though, as insufficient stomach acid can impair healthy digestion and the absorption of nutrients. The trick is to figure out how much acid suppression is just right to relieve symptoms without jeopardizing digestive health as a whole.

Infection with Helicobacter pylori

The spiral-shaped bacteria Helicobacter pylori has been found to play a significant role in the emergence of stomach ulcers. This bacterium invades the mucosal layer of the stomach, weakening it and increasing the stomach's vulnerability to the harmful effects of gastric acid. H. Worldwide, pylori infection is common and typically acquired in childhood. Although many people may carry the bacteria without showing any symptoms, in certain situations, it can cause ulcers and chronic inflammation.

Treatment of stomach ulcers frequently includes taking care of H. pylori infection with medication for antibiotics. Antibiotics and acid-suppressing drugs have been shown to work well together to eradicate the bacteria and accelerate ulcer healing. early identification of H. pylori infection is essential for prompt treatment and stopping the development of stomach ulcers. New approaches to treatment and tactics to counter H are still being researched. pylori, striving toward more focused and effective methods.

Stress and Lifestyle's Role

The onset and aggravation of stomach ulcers are mostly influenced by stress and lifestyle choices.

Although stress may not be a direct cause of ulcers, it can exacerbate symptoms and slow down the healing process. Prolonged stress causes physiological reactions that raise the risk of stomach ulcers by impairing immune system function and producing more gastric acid.

Managing stomach ulcers largely involves leading a healthy lifestyle. Making dietary decisions that minimize alcohol, smoke, and spicy food intake can also help soothe the lining of the stomach. Stress-reduction methods like relaxation exercises and meditation can improve general well-being and aid in the healing process.

Genetic Elements

Another element contributing to the susceptibility to stomach ulcers is genetics. People who have a family history of ulcers may be more likely to get them themselves. Genetic differences in the reaction to H or in the synthesis of mucosal protective substances.

ulcer susceptibility may be influenced by pylori infection.

Comprehending the hereditary aspects of gastric ulcers helps direct customized therapeutic strategies. hereditary testing can be used to identify people who are more vulnerable to certain hereditary vulnerabilities and to guide the development of specialized interventions. Furthermore, continuing research endeavors to decipher the complex genetic elements that contribute to ulcer development, hence facilitating the development of targeted medicines and preventive measures.

Finally, a thorough comprehension of the complex interactions between stomach acid, H. Effective treatment of stomach ulcers requires addressing the pylori infection, stress, lifestyle, and hereditary factors. The comprehensive care and prevention of this gastrointestinal ailment may benefit from the combination of medical interventions, lifestyle changes, and customized strategies based on genetic discoveries.

CHAPTER THREE

GETTING EXPERT ASSISTANCE
Consultation with a Healthcare Provider Is Important

It is crucial to seek professional assistance while managing the possible risk of stomach ulcers. Peptic ulcers, often known as stomach ulcers, are dangerous medical diseases that need to be carefully assessed and treated. It is important to consult a healthcare provider for several reasons.

First of all, since symptoms of stomach ulcers might overlap with other gastrointestinal problems, self-diagnosis and self-medication can be dangerous. To accurately determine whether stomach ulcers are present, a trained healthcare expert must evaluate the patient's medical history, examine the symptoms, and perform the required diagnostic tests. Ignoring or treating ulcers on your own without consulting a specialist might cause problems that worsen the condition and postpone necessary treatment.

Second, medical professionals possess the skills and information necessary to create a personalized treatment plan that meets each patient's unique needs. The intensity of ulcers varies, and each individual may have a different underlying cause. Patients can get tailored medical advice, prescription drugs, and lifestyle suggestions that address the underlying cause of their stomach ulcers by speaking with a healthcare professional. Seeking expert advice guarantees a thorough strategy for treating and eliminating stomach ulcers, resulting in more efficient and long-lasting outcomes.

In addition, medical professionals can keep an eye on how a patient is responding to treatment, make any required modifications, and deal with any side effects. To monitor the healing process and make well-informed decisions for the continued management of stomach ulcers, it is imperative to schedule routine follow-up appointments.

To guarantee the best possible outcome for those with stomach ulcers, it is crucial to consult with a healthcare provider for an accurate diagnosis, customized treatment programs, and continuing monitoring.

Examinations to Diagnose Stomach Ulcers:

Treatment for stomach ulcers must be administered with precision. Healthcare providers can confirm the existence of ulcers and assess their severity using a variety of diagnostic tests. One popular and very accurate diagnostic for identifying stomach ulcers is endoscopy. An endoscopy allows doctors to see into the digestive tract by passing a thin, flexible tube through the mouth and into the stomach lining. This enables medical personnel to examine ulcerations up close, obtain biopsies for additional examination, and gauge the degree of damage.

Furthermore, imaging tests like CT scans or X-rays can be used to detect ulcers and evaluate side effects including bleeding or perforation. The common cause of stomach ulcers, Helicobacter pylori infection, can also be diagnosed using blood tests. H. Analyzing blood samples for the presence of antibodies or antigens linked to the bacterium is known as pylori testing.

In addition, breath tests using urea are used to identify H. pylori. The patient consumes a urea solution tagged with a unique carbon atom during this test. Should H. Because Helicobacter pylori is present, it generates an enzyme that breaks down urea and releases carbon dioxide, which is detectable in breath.

In summary, a variety of diagnostic procedures enable medical professionals to precisely identify stomach ulcers, ascertain the underlying causes of these conditions, and customize treatment regimens for the best outcomes.

Choosing the Correct Specialist:

Selecting the appropriate specialist is a crucial first step on the road to recovery when battling stomach ulcers. Physicians who specialize in the diagnosis and treatment of digestive system illnesses, such as stomach ulcers, are known as gastroenterologists. These professionals have the knowledge and experience needed to handle the complexity of gastrointestinal problems and offer all-encompassing care.

A gastroenterologist can offer valuable advice because of their extensive understanding of the different causes of stomach ulcers. They can carry out comprehensive assessments, which may involve diagnostic testing, to determine the underlying cause of the ulcers. This could entail determining whether an infection with Helicobacter pylori is present, analyzing lifestyle choices, and taking into account any underlying medical issues that might be making the ulcers worse.

Moreover, gastroenterologists are knowledgeable about the most recent developments in gastrointestinal medicine, guaranteeing that patients receive state-of-the-art, scientifically supported care. Their particular focus makes it possible to manage stomach ulcers in a more targeted and nuanced manner, which improves results.

It is noteworthy that cooperation with other medical specialists can also be required, contingent upon the patient's general state of health and any comorbidities. For instance, to guarantee a comprehensive approach to care, a cardiologist may be consulted if the patient has cardiovascular problems.

In summary, selecting the appropriate specialist—a gastroenterologist in particular—is essential to receiving precise diagnosis, customized treatment regimens, and knowledgeable advice along the way to conquer stomach ulcers.

Questions to Put to Your Physician:

Asking relevant questions at your doctor's visits is a crucial aspect of being an active patient who wants to defeat stomach ulcers under professional guidance. Asking these questions can help you and your healthcare practitioner communicate openly and effectively while also providing a deeper understanding of your illness and treatment options.

To begin with, find out the details of your diagnosis. You will be better able to choose your course of therapy if you are aware of the kind, extent, and contributing factors of your stomach ulcers. Inquire about the outcomes of diagnostic procedures like endoscopies and blood tests, and ask questions about any unfamiliar medical terms or jargon.

Talk about possible treatments next. Consult your physician about the best course of action, which may include taking medication, changing your lifestyle, and, if required, undergoing surgery. Ask about the anticipated length of the course of treatment and any possible adverse effects from the prescription drugs. Your dedication to following the recommended regimen will be strengthened if you comprehend the reasoning behind every element of your treatment strategy.

Additionally, get advice on modifying your lifestyle to aid in the healing process and stop stomach ulcers from coming again. Long-term therapy success may depend critically on dietary changes, stress reduction strategies, and other lifestyle changes.

Talking about the schedule for monitoring and follow-up appointments is also crucial. Being aware of the evaluation standards for treatment outcomes and the frequency of check-ups will enable you to continue taking an active role in your health care.

Finally, don't be afraid to inquire about any possible issues or red flags that would need to be taken seriously right away. Protecting your health requires you to recognize warning signs and to know when to seek emergency medical attention.

In conclusion, asking meaningful questions of your healthcare provider proactively is crucial to effectively combating stomach ulcers under professional supervision. By fostering a collaborative partnership, open communication increases the likelihood of good treatment outcomes and gives you the power to actively engage in your care.

CHAPTER FOUR

TREATMENT OPTIONS
Medications for Stomach Ulcers

The first line of treatment for stomach ulcers is frequently medication designed to lower the stomach's excessive acidity, encourage healing, and ease symptoms. PPIs, or proton pump inhibitors, are frequently recommended because they stop the stomach lining's proton pump from producing acid. The ulcer can heal more successfully as a result of this decrease in acid production. H2 blockers are a different class of drugs that relieve symptoms and encourage ulcer healing by reducing the production of stomach acid. Antacids may also be suggested to counteract stomach acid and offer instant relief.

In situations where Helicobacter pylori (H. pylori) infection—a common bacterial infection associated with the formation of stomach ulcers—is the cause of the ulcer, antibiotics may be recommended. When acid-reducing drugs are used alongside antibiotics, the infection is eliminated and the healing process is sped up. To create a barrier that protects the ulcer from the corrosive effects of stomach acid and promotes healing, cytoprotective medicines like sucralfate may also be used.

People receiving medication-based treatment must carefully adhere to their recommended regimen and notify their healthcare provider of any side effects or concerns. For the best possible treatment results, the drug schedule may need to be reviewed and adjusted regularly.

Modifications to Diet and Lifestyle

A complete approach to managing stomach ulcers involves not just medication but also dietary and lifestyle changes. Patients are frequently recommended to cut back or avoid using certain substances, such as alcohol, tobacco, and nonsteroidal anti-inflammatory medicines (NSAIDs), as these might worsen the symptoms of ulcers. NSAIDs, such as ibuprofen and aspirin, can irritate the lining of the stomach and prevent ulcers from healing.

It's imperative to switch to a stomach-friendly diet. Usually, this entails eating more often and in smaller portions to lessen the strain on the digestive system. Steer clear of coffee, spicy, and acidic foods to reduce irritation to the ulcerated area. A diet high in fruits, vegetables, and whole grains supports the healing process and offers vital elements for general health.

Since stress can exacerbate ulcer symptoms, stress management practices like mindfulness meditation and deep breathing exercises are advised. Maintaining general well-being and assisting the body's inherent healing processes also heavily depends on getting enough sleep and exercising regularly.

Procedures Surgical

In cases when lifestyle changes and medicines fail to produce the intended outcomes or complications develop, surgical treatments for the treatment of stomach ulcers could be taken into consideration. Surgical alternatives include antrectomy, which includes removing the bottom section of the stomach where the majority of the acid is produced, and vagotomy, which involves severing the vagus nerve to minimize stomach acid production.

Emergency surgery can be required to seal the stomach wall perforation or stop the bleeding if an ulcer causes excessive bleeding. Minimally invasive surgeries, like laparoscopy, are frequently used in modern surgical techniques to reduce recovery time and postoperative problems.

People having surgical procedures should always be properly informed about the expected results, potential dangers, and benefits. Following surgery, with diet modifications and follow-up sessions, is essential to a full recovery.

Alternative and Supplemental Medical Practices

Some people look into complementary and alternative therapies in addition to traditional medical treatments as a way to enhance their ulcer management strategy. It is crucial to remember that these methods may or may not be beneficial, and using them should be reviewed with a healthcare provider.

Some people think that herbal medicines with anti-inflammatory and calming qualities, such as licorice and aloe vera, can help heal ulcers. But, care should be taken because these chemicals may worsen pre-existing medical issues or interfere with prescription drugs.

Some people find that alternative therapies like acupuncture and acupressure help treat ulcer symptoms and enhance general well-being. These methods entail stimulating particular body spots to promote the body's natural healing processes and reduce discomfort.

When integrating complementary and alternative medicines into a treatment plan for ulcers, patients must be transparent with their healthcare professionals. These methods ought to be seen as an addition to evidence-based medical care, not as a replacement for it.

To make sure that any alternative therapies selected are in line with the patient's overall health and treatment objectives, regular monitoring and consultation with healthcare professionals are imperative.

CHAPTER FIVE

NUTRITION AND DIET IN THE MANAGEMENT OF STOMACH ULCERS
Items to Add to Your Diet:

When creating a diet plan to treat stomach ulcers, foods that are healing and mild on the stomach lining must be carefully considered. It's important to choose foods that are readily digested and high in nutrients. Fruits like berries, apples, and bananas can add important vitamins and antioxidants to a diet. These fruits improve general health in addition to being easy on the stomach. When cooked to a soft texture, vegetables such as spinach, carrots, and zucchini provide a range of nutrients without exacerbating the symptoms of ulcers.

Fish, tofu, and skinless chicken are examples of lean protein sources that can be crucial to the healing process. Without putting an excessive amount of strain on the digestive system, these proteins supply the building blocks required for tissue healing. Furthermore, whole grains like oats, brown rice, and quinoa can provide a healthy amount of fiber and energy while also supporting digestive health and preventing ulcer symptoms. Yogurt and fermented foods include probiotics, which help maintain a balanced gut microbiota and promote healing.

It may be advantageous to include unsaturated fats from foods like almonds, avocados, and olive oil. These fats support healthy living and facilitate the absorption of nutrients. Finally, herbal teas that promote a quiet digestive environment, such as ginger or chamomile tea, can offer calming comfort.

Foods to Steer Clear of:

When it comes to controlling stomach ulcers, avoiding certain meals is equally as important as including others. Tomatoes, acidic fruits, and spicy meals should be avoided or consumed in moderation as they might irritate the lining of the stomach.

Due to their high acidity, citrus fruits—such as oranges and grapefruits—can aggravate ulcer symptoms and impede their healing.

Reduce your intake of fried and fatty meals as well, as these can exacerbate the formation of stomach acid and slow the healing of ulcers.

Because processed meats are high in chemicals and preservatives, they should not be included in a diet that is conducive to ulcers because they might cause pain and inflammation. Limiting caffeine and fizzy drinks can help control ulcers because they are known to increase the secretion of stomach acid.

Even though they may be appealing, sweets and sugary foods can impede the healing process by increasing inflammation. Pastries, chocolate, and candy should be avoided. Furthermore, it is imperative to restrict or completely avoid alcohol and tobacco consumption since they may hinder the stomach's healing process and elevate the likelihood of problems.

Strategies for Meal Planning:

Planning meals well is essential to controlling stomach ulcers. In addition to offering a more consistent supply of nutrients, eating smaller, more often meals throughout the day can help reduce the development of excessive amounts of stomach acid. Eating with full teeth facilitates digestion and eases the pressure on the stomach.

Keeping the macronutrient balance in each meal is crucial, involving a mix of complex carbohydrates, lean proteins, and healthy fats. In addition to promoting general health, this equilibrium guarantees a steady release of energy without taxing the digestive system.

Meal timing is similarly crucial. Eating the last meal of the day two or three hours before going to bed promotes healthy digestion and lowers the risk of acid reflux during the night. Since stress has been shown to worsen the symptoms of ulcers, making thoughtful eating choices during stressful times can also help promote improved digestive health.

The Value of Hydration

Maintaining general health and treating stomach ulcers both heavily depend on proper hydration. By keeping the stomach's mucosal lining well-hydrated, one can avoid the stomach from becoming overly acidic or irritable. Water also facilitates nutrient absorption and digestion, guaranteeing the body gets the building blocks it needs to repair.

As important as it is to stay hydrated, excessive intake of carbonated and caffeinated beverages should be avoided because they might aggravate and increase the formation of stomach acid. Choosing herbal teas can be calming to the digestive tract, especially if they contain anti-inflammatory ingredients like peppermint or chamomile.

Including foods high in water, such as cucumber, celery, and watermelon, in the diet helps stay hydrated and gives you extra nutrients. Individual hydration requirements must be taken into consideration, and fluid intake must be modified appropriately, taking physical activity, climate, and general health into account.

Keeping adequate fluids helps repair stomach ulcers and promotes the body's natural healing mechanisms. A thorough strategy for managing ulcers through diet and nutrition must include regular monitoring of hydration status and deliberate decision-making to prioritize water intake.

CHAPTER SIX

STRATEGIES FOR STRESS REDUCTION
Understanding How Stress Affects Stomach Ulcers:

One common element that greatly contributes to the onset and aggravation of stomach ulcers is stress. Effective care of stomach ulcers requires an understanding of the complex relationship between stress and these conditions. Stress chemicals like cortisol and adrenaline are released by the body as a natural reaction when a person is under stress.

These hormones may cause the production of more stomach acid, which damages the stomach's protective lining and fosters the development of ulcers. Furthermore, stress impairs immunity, which makes it harder for the body to fight off the Helicobacter pylori bacteria, which is frequently responsible for stomach ulcers.

The first step in putting stress management techniques into practice and lessening their effect on stomach ulcers is acknowledging these physiological reactions.

Methods of Relaxation:

When it comes to managing stress related to stomach ulcers, relaxation methods are essential for reestablishing bodily equilibrium and relieving stress. For example, deep breathing techniques can assist control of the autonomic nervous system, which lowers the release of stress chemicals and fosters relaxation. Including mindfulness meditation in daily routines is helpful since it helps people stay in the present moment and away from stressors that might lead to the development of ulcers. Another useful method for developing both physical and mental relaxation is progressive muscle relaxation, which is methodically tensing and then relaxing different muscle groups. These methods give people useful tools to proactively manage stress in addition to immediately addressing the physiological effects of stress.

Body-Mind Techniques:

A broad spectrum of holistic techniques that recognize the connection between mental and physical health are included in mind-body practices. For example, yoga integrates breathing exercises, meditation, and physical postures to promote mental and physical balance. Research indicates that consistent yoga practice can lower stress levels, strengthen the immune system, and improve general well-being, which makes it an effective strategy for treating stomach ulcers. Similar to this, tai chi provides a low-impact but efficient way to reduce stress with its flowing, soft movements and emphasis on breathing. By incorporating these mind-body techniques into daily life, one can help prevent stomach ulcers and provide the groundwork for long-term stress management.

Creating a Lifestyle of Resilience:

Developing a resilient lifestyle entails forming routines and actions that improve general health and the body's capacity to handle stress.

Resilience is mostly dependent on getting enough sleep, which helps the body heal and rebuild, making it more resilient to stress. Frequent exercise has been associated with lower stress levels and happier moods, both of which support resilient thinking. Furthermore, keeping a diet that is well-balanced and full of foods high in nutrients and antioxidants helps the body fight the damaging effects of stress on stomach ulcers. People can avoid and treat stomach ulcers by building resilience through these lifestyle choices, which will act as a buffer against the negative effects of stress.

CHAPTER SEVEN

HOLISTIC METHODS OF REMEDY
Including the Mind, Body, and Spirit Connection

Overcoming stomach ulcers necessitates a comprehensive strategy that extends beyond treating the physical symptoms. An essential component of holistic therapy is integrating the mind-body-spirit link. This method acknowledges the complex interactions that exist between spiritual, bodily, and mental health.

Stress has a major effect on digestive health and is frequently a contributing factor to stomach ulcers. Techniques like deep breathing exercises and mindfulness meditation help people feel calmer and more relaxed, which reduces stress. Those who practice mindfulness in the present moment can lessen mental pressures that could worsen symptoms of stomach ulcers.

In addition, cultivating emotional fortitude and a positive outlook is essential to the healing process. By enabling people to see a healthy, balanced stomach lining, techniques like guided imagery and visualization can help them have a more optimistic attitude toward their healing process. Understanding the relationship between the mind, body, and spirit motivates people to treat the underlying causes of their stomach ulcers, resulting in a more comprehensive and long-lasting healing process.

Supplements and Herbal Remedies

Herbal medicines and supplements are great companions in the field of holistic therapy for stomach ulcers. Plant-based remedies found in nature can be used in conjunction with traditional medical care. For example, aloe vera, which is well known for its anti-inflammatory qualities, can help repair ulcerated tissues and calm the digestive tract. In a similar vein, licorice root can be added to improve mucosal protection and lower stomach acid secretion due to its inherent anti-ulcer qualities.

Furthermore, certain nutrients are essential for maintaining digestive health. For instance, probiotics help the gut grow good bacteria, which supports a healthy microbiome that promotes healing. Zinc supplements also support immune system performance and tissue healing, strengthening the body's defenses against and recuperation from stomach ulcers. Combining carefully chosen herbal remedies with vitamins provides a comprehensive strategy that supports the body's natural healing processes while also addressing symptoms.

For Gut Health, Try Yoga and Meditation

Yoga and meditation emphasize the strong link between the mind and the gut and are therefore effective parts of a comprehensive approach to treating stomach ulcers. Particularly for the digestive system, yoga poses can improve blood flow to the abdominal organs, which can aid in the healing process and reduce inflammation. Yoga promotes a harmonic balance between the physical and mental components of well-being by encouraging attentive movement and breathing.

On the other side, people can use meditation as a method to develop inner calm and resilience in the face of the difficulties that stomach ulcers provide. For example, mindful eating meditations encourage deliberate and mindful consumption, enabling people to enjoy their food and enhance their digestion. In addition to aiding in physical healing, the comprehensive fusion of yoga and meditation gives people the tools they need to successfully negotiate the emotional and psychological aspects of their healing process.

Changes to a Holistic Lifestyle

Holistic therapy for gastric ulcers includes complete lifestyle modifications in addition to targeted interventions.

Dietary changes are crucial, with a focus on whole, nutrient-dense foods that promote intestinal health. Including a range of fruits, vegetables, and whole grains minimizes inflammatory triggers and supplies vital vitamins and minerals. Furthermore important for maintaining mucosal integrity and preventing issues connected to stomach acid is adequate hydration.

Lifestyle changes that go beyond diet include time management, prioritization, and healthy coping strategies, among other stress-reduction strategies. Frequent exercise that is customized to each person's abilities enhances general well-being and lowers stress. Getting enough sleep is also essential since it enables the body to go through the required healing processes that aid in the healing of stomach ulcers. Adopting a holistic lifestyle approach enables people to take an active role in their healing process and recognizes the interdependence of many areas of well-being.

CHAPTER EIGHT

AVOIDING THE RECURRENCE OF STOMACH ULCERS
Strategies for Long-Term Maintenance:

Preventing the recurrence of stomach ulcers requires the development of efficient long-term maintenance measures. A key component of this approach is living a lifestyle that promotes general digestive health. Keeping a balanced diet full of fiber, lean proteins, and healthy fats is part of this. Including probiotics in daily life can also help to maintain a healthy gut microbiota, which can improve digestion and lessen the risk of ulcers.

In addition, it is critical to control stress because long-term stress can aggravate ulcer symptoms and impede the healing process. Using stress-relieving methods like yoga, mindfulness, and consistent exercise can be essential parts of a long-term maintenance program.

Another important but frequently disregarded element is getting enough sleep. Maintaining a regular, peaceful sleep schedule promotes the body's natural healing processes and helps keep ulcers from coming back.

One of the most important aspects of long-term ulcer prevention is medication control. Proton pump inhibitors (PPIs) and H2 blockers are examples of prescription drugs that patients should take as directed to reduce stomach acid production and speed up the healing of ulcers. It is crucial to have regular meetings with healthcare specialists to assess the efficacy of drugs and make necessary adjustments.

Aftercare with Medical Professionals:

Maintaining follow-up treatment with medical professionals is essential in the fight against recurrent stomach ulcers. Following the initial diagnosis and course of therapy, follow-up visits enable medical staff to evaluate the patient's status, track the healing of ulcers, and spot any possible problems. Patients can talk about any persisting symptoms during these follow-up meetings, which enables prompt intervention and treatment plan modification.

During follow-up appointments, medical professionals may do diagnostic tests, such as endoscopies or imaging studies, to see the stomach lining and make sure ulcers are healing properly. Healthcare providers might decide whether to continue or change a patient's medication based on how well the patient responds to treatment.

These follow-up appointments also provide a forum for patient education. Healthcare professionals can assist patients with individualized advice on food decisions, stress reduction methods, and lifestyle changes. Open communication is essential for fostering a collaborative approach to ulcer prevention between patients and healthcare providers.

Observing and Identifying Warning Indications:

To stop stomach ulcers from recurring, it is essential to follow patients closely and recognize warning signals as soon as possible. Patients should be made aware of the signs of an ulcer relapse, which include bloating, nausea, vomiting, and persistent abdominal pain. Healthcare practitioners should be informed as soon as possible of any deviation from the usual.

It's also critical to be conscious of your triggers that could make ulcer symptoms worse. People ought to recognize and stay away from things like alcohol, hot foods, and some drugs that may irritate the lining of their stomachs.

Keeping a food journal and recording any associations between food choices and the start of symptoms can help identify trends and facilitate well-informed lifestyle modifications.

Furthermore, it's critical to self-check frequently for indicators of gastrointestinal bleeding, such as dark or bloody feces. Early detection of these warning indicators can help with prompt medical action and consequence avoidance. A thorough ulcer prevention plan must include patient empowerment through instruction in these monitoring approaches.

Formulating an Adaptive Preventive Strategy:

Developing a customized preventive strategy is crucial to addressing the distinct factors influencing each person's risk of recurrent stomach ulcers. A comprehensive strategy should be included in this plan, taking into account lifestyle choices, food preferences, and general health.

Healthcare professionals must conduct a thorough assessment as the first stage in developing a customized preventive plan. To determine certain risk factors and triggers, they will assess the patient's medical history, family history, and lifestyle choices. A personalized plan can be created using this data, including food suggestions, stress-reduction strategies, and an appropriate exercise schedule.

Dietary adjustments may involve avoiding well-known irritants, such as spicy foods and acidic drinks, and placing a greater emphasis on consuming items that support healthy digestion. It may be suggested to patients to space out their meals throughout the day to avoid extended episodes of stomach acidity. It's also important to drink enough water to support the digestive process and preserve the integrity of the mucosa.

The customized preventive strategy should include lifestyle changes as well as a timetable for routine diagnostic testing and follow-up visits. This proactive strategy enables continuous evaluation and modification of the preventive plan in response to the person's reaction and any changing risk factors.

In general, patient and healthcare-provider collaboration is essential to the effectiveness of a personalized preventive plan. An efficient and long-lasting plan to stop stomach ulcers from recurring is built on open communication, dedication to lifestyle modifications, and compliance with medical advice.

CHAPTER NINE

NAVIGATING CHALLENGES IN STOMACH ULCER MANAGEMENT
Handling Side Effects of Treatment:

Treatment for stomach ulcers frequently includes taking a mix of drugs to lower stomach acid, encourage healing, and address underlying issues. Although these treatments have the potential to be beneficial, patients may also have to deal with a variety of negative effects. Proton pump inhibitors (PPIs) and antibiotics are common drugs used to treat H. pylori infection. Sadly, side effects from these medications might include headaches, diarrhea, and nausea.

Working closely with a healthcare practitioner is one way to mitigate side effects. Occasionally, discomfort can be reduced by experimenting with other formulations or adjusting medicine dosages. In situations when adverse effects continue, patients are urged to be open and honest with their medical team.

This collaboration facilitates the development of a treatment plan that is more individualized and efficient.

Modifying one's lifestyle in addition to taking medicine can enhance conventional medical procedures. Dietary changes that could worsen symptoms, such as avoiding hot or acidic meals, may be investigated by patients. Incorporating stress-reduction methods into daily life, such as yoga or mindfulness, can also improve general well-being and possibly minimize discomfort associated with treatment.

Handling the Psychological and Emotional Aspects:

The treatment of stomach ulcers affects people emotionally and psychologically in addition to physically. Increased tension and worry may result from the chronic nature of the illness and the possibility of periodic flare-ups. People could struggle with worries about how it would affect their relationships, daily activities, and quality of life in the long run.

Holistic care is necessary to address these psychological and emotional components. By including mental health assistance in the whole treatment plan, patients might gain more self-efficacy in managing their issues.

Counselors or psychologists with experience in chronic illness might offer helpful strategies for handling stress and negotiating the emotional challenges of having a stomach ulcer.

Additionally, support groups are a priceless tool for anyone coping with the psychological effects of stomach ulcers. Understanding and a sense of community are fostered by interacting with people who have gone through similar things. By sharing triumphs, offering sympathetic support, and exchanging coping mechanisms, patients can form a network that lessens the isolation that sometimes accompanies long-term conditions.

A strong support network is frequently necessary for patients and their caregivers to successfully navigate the challenges associated with managing stomach ulcers. A chronic illness affects not only the person with the diagnosis but also friends and family who may have to provide care.

It's critical to establish clear channels of communication within the support system. A foundation of understanding is established by having candid and open conversations regarding the difficulties in managing stomach ulcers, treatment options, and expectations. By keeping caregivers informed and connected, this communication helps guarantee that they can offer appropriate support.

Caregivers should also put their well-being first. Caring for someone who has a chronic disease can be mentally and physically exhausting. Caregivers must seek out respite, whether in the form of support groups, therapy, or just taking time out to refuel, to preserve their health and continue to be able to offer continuous support.

Overcoming Typical Obstacles:

Managing stomach ulcers is not without its difficulties; patients frequently run across problems that call for careful planning. One major obstacle is the requirement for lifestyle adjustments, which can be challenging to regularly follow and include food adjustments and stress management.

One important technique for overcoming these challenges is education. Patients can take an active role in their health by being empowered with full knowledge about the significance of following treatment programs, making lifestyle adjustments, and identifying early indicators of difficulties. In this educational process, healthcare providers are essential in ensuring that patients are knowledgeable and capable of making wise decisions.

Obstacles may also arise from financial concerns, especially for individuals who lack sufficient insurance coverage. It is essential that patients have access to the drugs and medical treatments they require, and healthcare professionals can work with patients to find affordable alternatives or support services.

Moreover, overcoming barriers to stomach ulcer treatment requires constant monitoring and follow-up. Frequent check-ins with medical professionals enable treatment regimens to be modified in response to changing patient demands and aid in the early detection of possible problems. Open communication about challenges is encouraged among patients, which promotes teamwork in overcoming barriers and maximizing long-term results.

CHAPTER TEN

INSPIRATIONAL JOURNEYS AND SUCCESS STORIES
Actual Accounts of People Who Overcame Stomach Ulcers:

When it comes to health issues, stomach ulcers are a powerful foe. Stomach ulcer recovery is frequently characterized by resiliency, tenacity, and an unwavering dedication to well-being. One person who overcame this illness describes the early days of unbearable suffering, the ambiguity around the diagnosis, and the ensuing search for a viable cure.

The road to recovery developed via teamwork with physicians, dietary changes, and lifestyle improvements. The person discusses the emotional rollercoaster of failures and achievements, illuminating the psychological and physical costs associated with managing stomach ulcers.

These actual events provide evidence of the human spirit's ability to persevere and overcome extreme health obstacles.

Statements from People Who Overcame Stomach Ulcers:

Testimonials from individuals who have conquered stomach ulcers provide a glimmer of hope to those facing comparable struggles. These testimonies go into great detail on the individual's battle with stomach ulcers, highlighting the critical role that professional advice played in their eventual recovery. The stories emphasize how crucial it is to have a customized treatment plan that addresses stress management, dietary modifications, and medication management.

Testimonials highlight the need for emotional support from family, friends, and healthcare professionals in addition to the clinical side. By sharing their personal stories, people debunk the myth that treating stomach ulcers is only a physical challenge and demonstrate the life-changing power of taking a holistic approach to wellness. For people looking for comfort and direction in their struggles with stomach ulcers, these testimonies serve as a constant source of inspiration.

Takeaways and Inspirational Realizations:

Although overcoming stomach ulcers is a difficult road, it also offers invaluable life lessons. Survivors frequently consider the lessons learned from their experience, providing insightful advice to those who are traveling a similar route. These people impart knowledge gleaned from personal experience, covering topics such as the value of proactive healthcare management and the contribution of stress reduction to the healing process.

Motivational insights explore the mental adjustments required to overcome obstacles, adopt a positive perspective, and develop resilience. Lessons learned touch on the connection between mental and emotional health and the healing process, going beyond the physical domain.

The stories encourage people to take a holistic approach to their health and acknowledge the mutually reinforcing link between lifestyle decisions and general well-being.

Motivation for the Upcoming Journey:

When people go out on their path to overcome stomach ulcers, a support system is essential. Seasoned survivors and those who have made it through this difficult terrain successfully offer words of wisdom to lift the spirits of others who are still in the process of healing. Encouragement places a strong emphasis on the value of endurance, patience, and the slow nature of healing. People talk about the importance of self-care and exhort people to pay attention to their health and listen to their bodies. Beyond the physical components of recovery, the encouragement emphasizes the mental toughness needed to confront the unknowns of a health journey. The community of conquerors creates a sense of togetherness among those still navigating the complex terrain of stomach ulcer recovery by providing encouraging comments that inspire hope.

CHAPTER ELEVEN

SELF-EMPOWERMENT FOR A WELL-BEING FUTURE
Taking Responsibility for Your Health

One of the most important steps in beating stomach ulcers is taking control of your health. It entails taking a proactive stance when it comes to comprehending and taking care of your well-being. Getting expert advice is the most important thing to do. Speaking with medical professionals and specialists can help you learn more about the causes, symptoms, and customized treatment options for stomach ulcers.

Additionally, self-education is essential to managing your health. You can make more informed lifestyle decisions if you are aware of the causes of stomach ulcers, which include bacterial infections, stress, and certain drugs. This could entail changing your nutrition, learning stress-reduction strategies, and starting a regular exercise regimen. You take an active role in your recovery by taking an active interest in your health.

Maintaining your health also involves getting regular checkups. Regular tests to monitor your health enable early detection and action, preventing complications related to stomach ulcers. Forming a collaborative relationship with your healthcare practitioner facilitates transparent communication, guaranteeing your active participation in treatment and general well-being decision-making.

Developing a Strategy for Holistic Well-Being

Developing a holistic approach to well-being is essential for a thorough strategy to combat stomach ulcers. This entails attending to the mental and emotional as well as the physical manifestations of health issues. For example, stress plays a big role in the onset and aggravation of stomach ulcers.

Including stress-reduction practices in your daily routine, such as yoga, meditation, and mindfulness, can support a comprehensive approach to well-being.

An important aspect of treating stomach ulcers is nutrition. A healthy, ulcer-friendly diet helps promote healing and stave against recurrence. This can mean including foods that support a healthy digestive tract and avoiding foods that are too spicy or acidic. A nutritionist consultation can offer individualized nutritional advice catered to your unique requirements and interests.

Additionally, developing a support system is critical to emotional health. Making connections with loved ones, friends, or support groups can offer shared experiences, understanding, and encouragement. Developing a holistic approach to well-being entails understanding how mental and physical health are intertwined, enabling a more thorough and successful management of stomach ulcers.

Promoting and Raising Awareness

Educating others about stomach ulcers and engaging in advocacy are essential steps in empowering oneself for a healthier future. Becoming an advocate helps dispel the stigma around gastrointestinal disorders and promotes candid discussions about digestive health. This entails speaking about your personal experiences, taking part in initiatives to raise awareness, and advocating for education regarding stomach ulcers.

Informing people about the symptoms, risk factors, and preventative measures associated with stomach ulcers is another way to spread awareness. This information promotes a culture of early diagnosis and intervention and gives people the confidence to take proactive measures for their digestive health. There are many ways to advocate, such as by taking part in local events or using social media to provide resources and information.

Additionally, promoting financial increases and policy modifications in the area of gastrointestinal health has a wider effect. You may help create a supportive atmosphere for people with stomach ulcers and other digestive illnesses by actively interacting with lawmakers, the public, and healthcare organizations.

Going Forward with Self-Assuredness

Taking control of your health, developing a comprehensive plan for your well-being, and raising awareness are the final steps toward moving forward with confidence. Positivity, following a customized treatment plan, and bodily awareness are the keys to managing stomach ulcers with confidence.

Retaining confidence requires setting reasonable objectives and acknowledging minor accomplishments along the way. Understanding that treating stomach ulcers is a journey and that improvement may occur gradually is crucial. Being physically well is just one aspect of confidence; other aspects include developing resiliency and flexibility in the face of adversity.

Maintaining contact with your medical group and support system also gives you a sense of security and assurance, which boosts your confidence in the treatment of stomach ulcers. Taking part in joyful and fulfilling activities enhances general well-being and cultivates an optimistic attitude toward the future.

In summary, taking charge of your health and moving forward with confidence is a dynamic process that calls for ongoing self-care, an optimistic outlook, and active involvement in your recovery. It is evidence of your tenacity and dedication to leading a happy, healthy life despite the difficulties caused by stomach ulcers.